Francesca Cesari and Lucia Wilson reserve the right to be identified as the photographer and writer of the work.

Lucia Wilson and Francesca Cesari are the co-editors and co-owners of the work.

© 2020 Francesca Cesari and Lucia Wilson

Cover photographs by Francesca Cesari

ISBN NO. 9798 3766 93742

Maymyo Publications

With heartfelt thanks

We want to thank our volunteer strabismus patients, Marilena, Anna Maria and Paul for their time, their patience, and their invaluable contribution to this book. Their commitment to helping raise the profile of strabismus is deeply appreciated.

We also want to offer our grateful thanks to Dr Silvia Riva, Dr Giovanni Battista Marcon and Mr Saurabh Jain who so generously contributed their expert knowledge and experience to work with us to shine a light on this poorly understood eye condition, its impact on patients and with a unified aim of making life better for all strabismus patients.

Many thanks, grazie mille, Lucia and Francesca.

Contents

***

1. Introduction

Face to Face with Strabismus is an international collaboration with a public engagement mission. It is the joint creation of photographer, Francesca Cesari in Bologna, and writer, Lucia Wilson, in London. Lucia is a former strabismus patient.

In association with leading eye surgeons, Mr Saurabh Jain of the Royal Free Hospital, London and Dr Giovanni Battista Marcon, a consultant ophthalmologist specialising in strabismus based in Bassano del Grappa, Vicenza, and Dr Silvia Riva, psychologist at Dottorelondon and a senior lecturer at St Mary's University, the team have sought to explore how strabismus impacts the lives of those with this poorly understood eye condition. They have also considered the reasons why strabismus patients are not always given the support they deserve.

Through photography and interviews with strabismus patients, Marilena, Anna Maria and Paul, the human story of strabismus is revealed.

Lucia has also shared her own experience with strabismus, as well as the story behind the diptych created with Francesca Cesari, which grew out of her frustration with the diplopia caused by strabismus. This unique image was a catalyst for the creation of the wider project, Face to Face, in 2020. Face to Face with Strabismus has evolved from their original concept.

Issues on the theme of self-perception, both visually and psychologically, are examined with psychologist, Dr Silvia Riva. Francesca Cesari provides a photographer's perspective following her photographic work with the patients and through her role as co-editor with Lucia Wilson.

As a result of their research, the discussions with the experts and interviews with patients, certain observations have come to light which demonstrate how strabismus (which is also referred to as a squint) has been obscured by confusion. Words Matter, written by Lucia Wilson, illustrates the source of this confusion. The section, No Joke, discusses how strabismus is often trivialised, even mocked.

Through the creation of this book, the team are endeavouring to shine a much-needed light on strabismus.

2. Living with Strabismus

- Marilena Bedin

- Anna Maria Bedin

- Paul Boyce

MARILENA

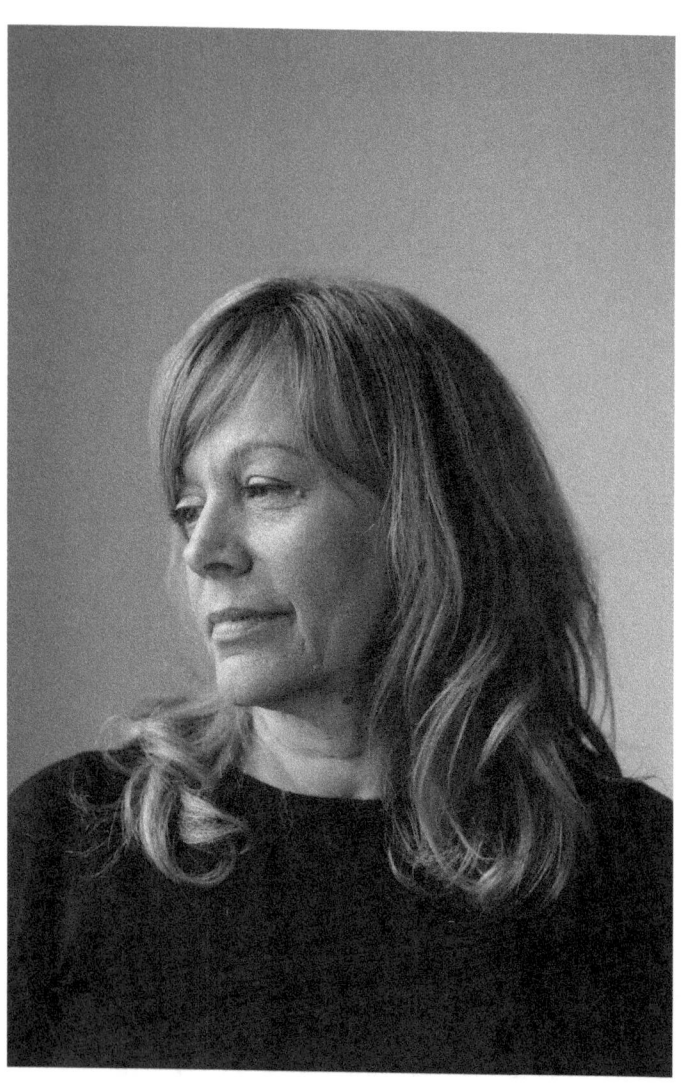

Marilena Bedin is a former strabismus patient from Rovigo, Italy.

Marilena is the sister of Anna Maria, also a strabismus sufferer who, at the time of her interview, was awaiting strabismus surgery.

Question1. Marilena, have you always had problems with your eyesight, other eye conditions besides strabismus? If so, can you tell us more?

Marilena:

I was probably born with myopia problems, my paternal grandfather was almost blind, my aunts very short-sighted, I am the seventh daughter: 6 women and 1 man, we are practically divided in half: 4 short-sighted, 3 without vision problems.

It was only at the age of 12 that my violin teacher realized that to look at the right page I turned my head completely, He called my parents and from there began my adventure with visual problems. I already knew it in my heart, but I didn't say anything to anyone, because I was ashamed.

Eye examination: high myopia on the right and myopia on the left, despite wearing glasses it did not correct my vision because the difference was so great. At 19 I started to use rigid contact lenses.

Question 2. Please tell us about your experience with strabismus - when did it first start? A) What symptoms did you have? B) How did it make you feel?

Marilena:

At the age of 40 I was advised by my ophthalmologist the possibility of removing the lenses (by then it was difficult to bear them all day) and I was operated on. I had cataract surgery on the right eye, then the left eye... with the intervention of "radial keratotomy".

This removed the myopia, leading me to the vision of 10 diopters, "paradise". This, however, slowly led me to an amblyopia, the right eye was falling asleep, and to the internal converging strabismus; sometimes I saw double but not always. The problems of acceptance of my "particular" gaze were making themselves felt.

Question 3. How did strabismus affect your daily life (compared to life before you had the

condition)? Did it affect a) your work? b) your quality of life? c) your interactions with family and friends? d) Do you have any experiences you would like to share?

Marilena:
Strabismus has greatly influenced my life, even if people did not point it out to me, I tried in every way to hide this defect even with a wrong posture, my head tilted. I smile at the thought of my hairdresser who tried in vain to put my head straight. I kept saying to myself that it was my characteristic, but if someone looked me straight in the eye, I felt very uncomfortable.

Question 4. Did you feel supported in managing your eye condition/was it easy to access help? a) via your GP or your hospital in Italy? B) via social services, for practical support/benefits? c) A support group?

Marilena:

Every year given my pathology, I underwent a thorough eye examination and every time I punctually
asked my doctor, Dr Camellin, to "solve the problem".
in 2017, I insisted so much that he decided to intervene surgically, as soon as I had my operation everything seemed resolved, even if apparently, I remember that when I put on make-up, I saw that the eye was brought too far inside. Once again, I wanted to lie to myself telling myself that everything was fine. Last December (2021) I went back to my ophthalmologist making the usual request once again, "please doctor please operate on me again".... I just need a dream for a few months. After a week, my ophthalmologist phoned me and referred me (God bless him) to Dr. Marcon. My current ophthalmologist Dr. Camellin Massimo is the best for my problems, but he recognized the utmost professionalism of his colleague Dr. Marcon.

Question 5. Do you feel that strabismus is taken seriously by a) those in your immediate circle – family/friends/colleagues? b) In the wider world?

Marilena:

Strabismus is not taken seriously at all, it is considered a physical defect, such as a crooked nose or a big belly etc, just a minor thing.. not so I can assure you.

Question 6: Did you receive treatment such as Botox injections? Or was surgery the main treatment? Can you say a bit more about this?

Marilena:

The surgery was the only treatment received.

Question 7. Are there any aids or tips that helped you manage day to day while you waited for surgery? For example, did prism spectacles help?
In my own case, double vision (diplopia) made me extremely nervous in different situations, for example, when going down a set of stairs, I developed a method of feeling for the back of each stair with the heel of my foot before progressing. I

became anxious, especially after several accidents caused by my double vision. Did you develop things like that to help you to manage?

Marilena:

After the surgery that took place in November 2017 (carried out by Dr. Camellin in Rovigo), I began to see double, I commanded myself to see only one figure or at worst, I closed one eye, and then slowly I got used to it. I have never had particular problems in the sense of falls or accidents due to double vision, having one predominant eye, at worst I closed the other eye.

Question 8. How did you feel about your self-image? For example, how did you feel about your reflection in a mirror?
a) Did your reflection alter as with some patients who have diplopia (double vision) which is caused by their strabismus? b) Were you very conscious of your

eyes being misaligned and did that make you uncomfortable with other people? c) Do you have any experiences to share?

Marilena:

When I looked in the mirror, I noticed precisely the non-alignment, so I got very close and it seemed to me that then the defect was not so relevant, as soon as I moved away "Oh, Gosh! Complete crisis." Sometimes, to make a joke some friend, laughing, twisted his eyes (in front of me). I was very angry, I felt really teased,
even if I'm honest no one ever made me feel really bad about it. Indeed, they often told me that it was my characteristic, but I was not well, I didn't feel at ease.

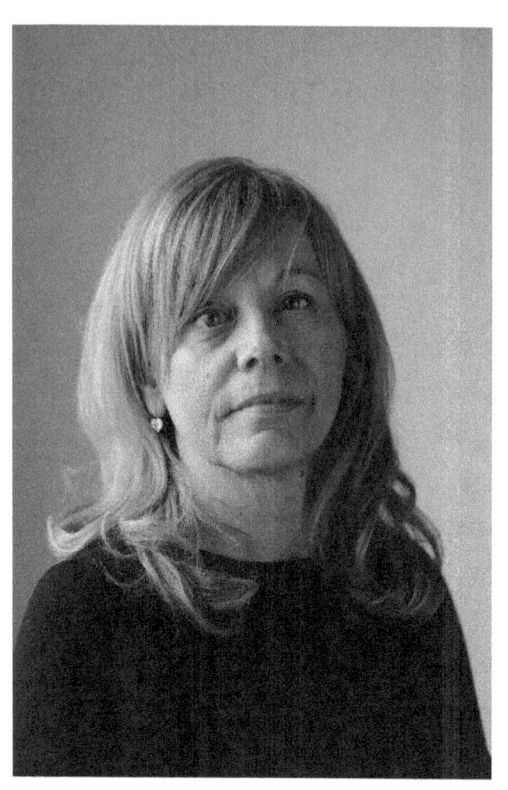

Question 9. Did you feel differently about your self-image once you developed strabismus? a) Did you find that others looked at you differently?

Marilena:

I can say that the real strabismus began to be present...I realized it at a mature age let's say around 40 years. Before that, perhaps it was hidden by the look - 'always suffering and tired' of those who continuously wear contact lenses. I repeat, maybe yes, others had noticed it (the strabismus) for some time, but maybe, so as not to hurt me, they never pointed it out. Perhaps they thought about it, because after the last operation, the compliments were many, and only at that moment they were sincere (and now I speak only of the aesthetic improvement).

Question 10. Did you describe yourself as disabled? Did you use the term? a) Were you comfortable to be described as disabled?

Marilena:

I can tell you that just after 40 I was subjected to a visit by the occupational doctor (a woman). I am an administrative employee and I work in front of a video terminal 8 hours a day. As soon as she saw me, she immediately asked me, I also remember in a not very tender tone, if by chance when I was born, my mother remembered some trauma from childbirth, because I was all asymmetrical. She described me as if I were a "monster"; from there my ordeal was born, I began to look at myself with different eyes. although I admit it (I am not vain) I often receive compliments for my physical appearance .... nevertheless, I have never felt disabled, I have a normal driving licence, and I am professionally fulfilled. My only goal: the problem had to be solved.

Question 11. How are you feeling about being photographed for our project? Excited? Nervous? A) Did you feel differently about being photographed once you developed strabismus?

B) Are you happier to be photographed now you no longer have strabismus?

Marilena:

Oh my God, photography!!!! Maximum taboo (it is too honest), never before did I want to be photographed. Even if I admit it even today, I do not like that others photograph me, I take selfies and I can say that up to this point I have not noticed "anomalies", but I am sincere, for now I am happy. But I am still ready for a relapse, I say to myself " but yes .... In Bassano, fortunately, there is Dr. Marcon – no matter how bad things get, he can fix it..... I don't resist if I see someone taking photographs... but I feel terror even today.

Question 12. Is there anything that I haven't asked you about your experience of strabismus that you

would like to add to this discussion? If yes, please feel free to share this below.

Marilena:

I can add that beyond the physical aspect to which we women aspire, my field of vision is much improved, now I no longer see double even if I have been warned that this could happen. Since May 23 (the date of the operation that Dr. Marcon did for me) I see better on

the right without turning my head. My strabismus was not corrected completely, unfortunately, due to the diversity also of the eyeball of the eye *and*, as already anticipated with high myopia - maybe Dr. Marcon will be more specific about the details of this - but today I'm happy. I do not suffer, I look others in the eyes, and I no longer hear myself say, sorry but "that eye" seems a bit strange. I don't know if this "miracle" will last for a long time, forever, for a year, a month, for a lifetime... but just knowing that there is a solution, everything seems easier. I want to recommend this operation to everyone... Certainly there's a bit of initial pain (but not so much in truth) a few days of rest and then away ... stronger than before.

This is a close verbatim translation from Italian to English using translation software.

Photography of Marilena Bedin by Francesca Cesari

ANNA MARIA

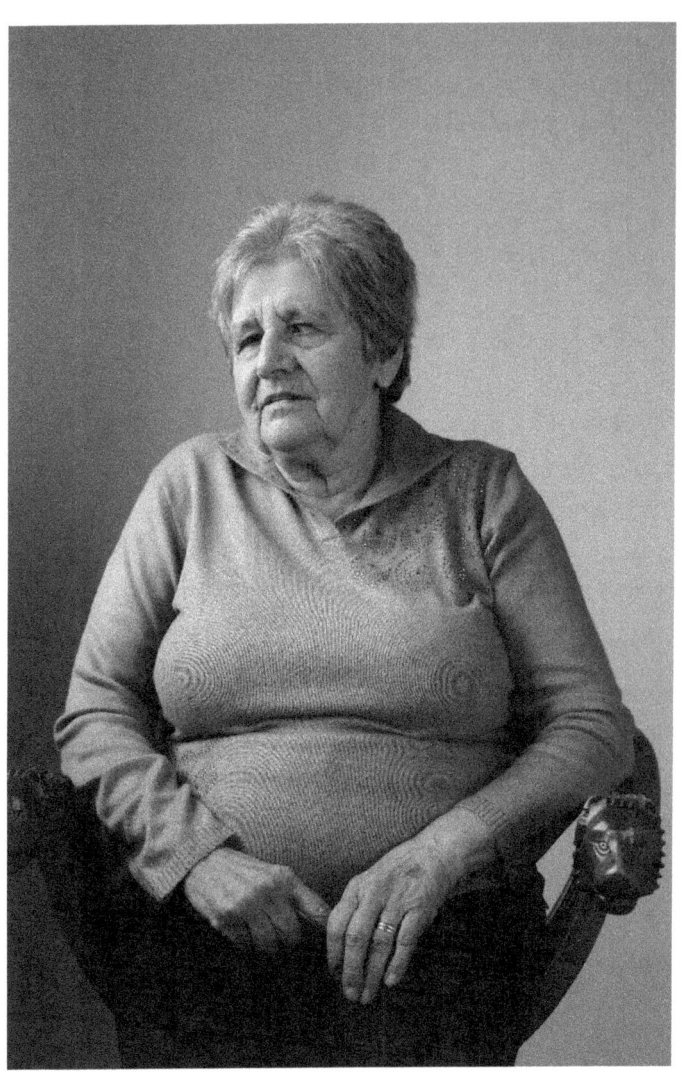

Anna Maria Bedin is a strabismus patient from Rovigo, Italy; she is the sister of Marilena Bedin, also a former strabismus patient.

At the time of this interview, Anna Maria was awaiting strabismus surgery.

Question 1. Have you always had problems with your eyesight, other eye conditions besides strabismus? If so, can you tell us more?

Anna Maria:

I was born short-sighted, I am 76 years old I was the first daughter of two young parents who slowly saw 6 more children arrive (6 females and 1 male, to be precise). My grandfather and paternal aunts already suffered from high myopia, and an aunt - I do not remember from what age, but she was also cross-eyed.

Question 2. Please tell us about your experience with strabismus - when did it first start? a) What symptoms do you have? b) How does it make you feel?

Anna Maria:

I do not remember but I have confirmation from the few photos taken on the occasion of weddings or ceremonies to confirm I have had problems with strabismus before adulthood, certainly after 40 years, after cataract surgery on both eyes, I had no particular problems, my life continued to maintain my usual rhythms.

Question 3. How does strabismus affect your daily life (compared to life before you had the condition)? Does it affect a) Your work? b) Your quality of life? c) Your interactions with family and friends? D) Do you have any experiences you would like to share?

Anna Maria:

I have not had an easy life - a very bad accident happened to my son just over sixteen years old and there was the loss of my husband at the age of 49, so there was no time to think about my problems, and the strabismus honestly seemed to me only an "aesthetic defect".

There was no time; one eye troubled me more than the other also for the difference in myopia, meanwhile the years have passed, and I no longer considered it important to "correct" this defect of mine. I am this way and that's it - nobody has ever made me feel uncomfortable because of it or made me feel "different", even if in my heart, I was unhappy. I suffered, I avoided looking in the mirror, but I encouraged my younger sister, younger than about twenty years, who began to have the same problem, fortunately only in one eye, to look for a solution.

Question 4. Do you feel supported in managing your eye condition, was it easy to access help? a) via

your GP or your hospital in Italy?   b) via social services, for practical support/benefits? c) A support group?

Anna Maria:

No one has ever advised me to find a solution, not even my ophthalmologist, to be honest. My sister who in the meantime was inquiring for herself, tried to inquire for me, but in my case, there was talk of strabismus "fixed" and therefore not curable.

Question 5. Do you feel that strabismus is taken seriously by a) those in your immediate circle – family/friends/colleagues? b) In the wider world?

Anna Maria:

Strabismus is not taken seriously, no one imagines the suffering it causes.

Question 6 Do you receive treatment such as Botox injections? Or is your upcoming surgery the main

treatment? Can you say a bit more about this?

Anna Maria:

Dr. Marcon was recommended to me by my ophthalmologist, Dr. Camellin. Unfortunately, during the last check-up, he could not even check the eye because it was slowly going more and more towards the inside and my vision consequently fails. I was not very convinced of the operation, at my age, but I cannot decide otherwise. I am hopeful for the intervention that will be carried out on 21/11/2022, I don't expect aesthetic improvements, but I cross my fingers to see more.

Question 7. Are there any aids or tips that help you manage day to day while you wait for surgery for example, do prism spectacles help? In my own case, double vision (diplopia) made me extremely nervous in different situations, for example, when

going down a set of stairs, I developed a method of feeling for the back of each stair with the heel of my foot before progressing. I became anxious, especially after several accidents caused by my double vision. Have you developed things like that to help you to manage?

Anna Maria:
I have never used prism glasses and any other aid, I have never seen double, also because from one eye I see only a few diopters.

Question 8. How do you feel about your self-image? For example, how do you feel about your reflection in a mirror? a) Has your reflection altered as with some patients who have diplopia (double vision) which is caused by their strabismus? b) Are you very conscious of your eyes being misaligned and does that make you uncomfortable with other people? c) Do you have any experiences to share?

Anna Maria:

I absolutely avoid looking in the mirror, and if I talk to someone I look down, I feel uncomfortable, I don't accept myself.

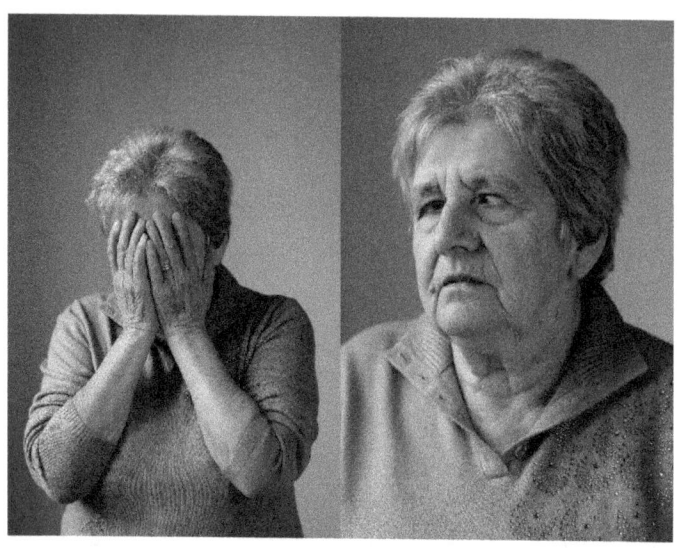

Question 9. Do you feel differently about your self-image since you developed strabismus? A) Do you find that others look at you differently?

Anna Maria:

I repeat I do not look in the mirror, I absolutely avoid it.

Question 10. Do you describe yourself as disabled? Do you use the term? a) Are you comfortable to be described as disabled?

Anna Maria:
I don't feel disabled, I don't have a driving licence, not because of strabismus but because of myopia.

Question 11 How are you feeling about being photographed for our project? Excited? Nervous? A) Do you feel differently about being photographed since you developed strabismus? B) Do you think you will be happier to be photographed once you no longer have strabismus?

Anna Maria:
I avoid photography, my loved ones know it and if I really can't escape, I get behind the others so that I am less visible in the photo..

Question 12. Is there anything that I haven't asked you about your experience of strabismus that you would like to add to this discussion? If yes, please feel free to share this below.

Anna Maria:

I do not think that the operation completely solves the aesthetic problem, but I do not care, honestly I have been living with this problem for years and I really

hope to see better. Above all I would like to be able to be autonomous to get by, for me the problem is that I no longer see well, not that I had a clear and normal vision before, but it was enough for me.

This is a close verbatim translation from Italian to English using translation software.

Photography of Anna Maria Bedin by Francesca Cesari

PAUL

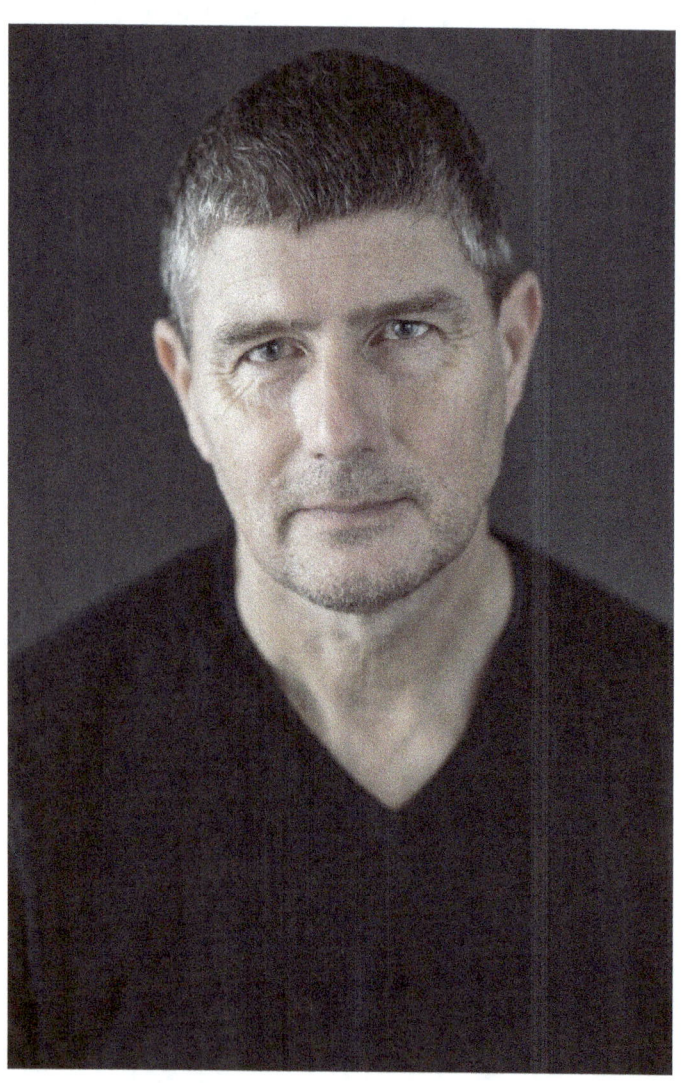

Paul Boyce is a former strabismus patient living in London. Paul was diagnosed with fourth nerve palsy when his squint was investigated. His strabismus differed in its presentation to that of the patients from Italy, and from Lucia's own experience. Paul was under the care of Mr Saurabh Jain.

Question 1. Have you always had problems with your eyesight, other eye conditions besides strabismus? If so, can you tell us more?

Paul
Up until 2015 (when I was in my 40s) I hadn't noticed any real problems with my eyes, but I did get reading glasses in 2013.

Question 2. Please tell us about your experience with strabismus - when did it first start? a) What symptoms did you have? b) How did it make you feel?

Paul

a. I didn't notice that I was having any symptoms. However, in 2015 my wife and children first noticed my left eye would go to the right and up and almost disappear. Also, my GP spotted this when I visited him for a different health matter.

In addition to the squint – I have always called it a squint, not strabismus – it was pointed out to me that it was becoming obvious (although not to me) that I was tilting my head a lot. I also had double vision sometimes, not all the time.

b. To be honest it didn't make me feel any different, but now I look back on it, I think I was also a bit in denial.

Question 3. How did strabismus affect your daily life (compared to life before you had the condition)? Did it affect a) Your work? b) Your quality of life?

c) Your interactions with family and friends? d) Do you have any experiences you would like to share?

Paul

a) I was working as a printer but had stopped working because of an injury (not connected with strabismus).

In spite of the symptoms I was having, I managed, it didn't impact my ability to do my job.

My quality of life was not affected because over time my body had adapted to this condition which is called fourth nerve palsy. Until my diagnosis I was unaware there was a problem.

b) Until I was diagnosed, family and friends would make remarks and say "Dad/Paul stop looking at us in a strange way."

I would say I didn't know I was and, according to my family and friends, I would get quite defensive.

Question 4. Did you feel supported in managing your eye condition/was it easy to access help? a) via your GP or your hospital? b) via social services, for practical support/benefits? C) A support group?

Paul

a. I saw my GP on another matter when he noticed something wrong with my left eye. He referred me to

a local eye clinic who then in turn referred me to Mr. Jain. I was diagnosed with fourth nerve palsy and Mr Jain recommended surgery. My treatment throughout this whole experience and even now has been amazing and without fault.

Question 5. Do you feel that strabismus is taken seriously by a) those in your immediate circle family/friends/colleagues? b) In the wider world?

Paul

a. Because my squint didn't affect my day-to-day life people around me didn't realise I had a serious eye condition and were unaware of the term strabismus.

Question 6. Did you receive treatment such as Botox injections? Or was surgery the main treatment? Can you say a bit more about this?

Paul

My main treatment was strabismus surgery on the 13/11/17 for left eye, fourth nerve palsy.

Question 7 Are there any aids or tips that helped you manage day to day while you waited for surgery? For example, did prism spectacles help? In my case, double vision (diplopia) made me extremely nervous in different situations, for example, when going down a set of stairs, I developed a method of feeling for the back of each stair with the heel of my foot before progressing. I became anxious, especially after several accidents caused by my double vision. Did you develop things like that to help you to manage?

Paul

As I said earlier, I didn't recognise that I had a problem and my body compensated unknowingly, resulting in a quite pronounced head tilt at times. Before and after surgery I would blink once or twice to refocus to lose the double vision which I am still doing now. Before my diagnosis, I thought this was due to tiredness and poorly lit environments.

Question 8. How did you feel about your self-image? For example, how did you feel about your reflection in a mirror? a) Did your reflection alter as with some patients who have diplopia (double vision) which is caused by their strabismus? b) Were you very conscious of your eyes being misaligned and did that make you uncomfortable with other people? C) Do you have any experiences to share?

Paul

a. Before and after surgery when I looked in the mirror, I just saw myself, no difference just me.

As I mentioned earlier, I was a bit defensive when others said that I was looking at them in a funny way, if they pointed out that my eyes were not straight.

b) No.

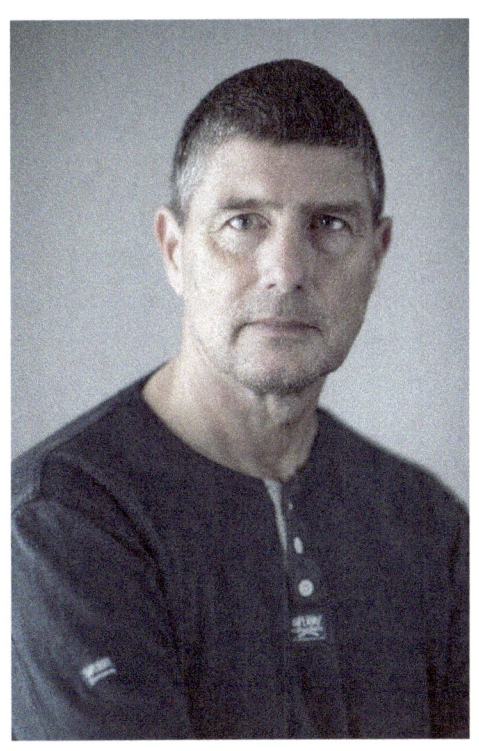

Question 9. Did you feel differently about your self-image once you developed strabismus? a) Did you find that others looked at you differently?

Paul

No, I have always been ok about the way I looked.

Question 10. Did you describe yourself as disabled? Did you use the term? a) Were you comfortable to be described as disabled?

Paul

It never crossed my mind that my squint was a disability because it didn't affect my day-to-day life. However, having a squint is not a trivial problem and I am very glad that I had my surgery.

Question 11. How are you feeling about being photographed for our project? Excited? Nervous? a) Did you feel differently about being photographed once you developed strabismus? b) Are you happier to be photographed now you no longer have strabismus?

Paul

I am feeling ok about being photographed.

a. No.

Question 12. Is there anything that I haven't asked you about your experience of strabismus that you would like to add to this discussion? If yes, please feel free to share this below.

Paul

No, I am happy to be involved in your book.

Photography of Paul Boyce by Remy Hunter

3.Lucia's strabismus story

In this section, I want to describe what it was like for me to live with strabismus, the symptoms, the impact on daily life and my general wellbeing.

I also want to share a number of observations regarding my experience to help shine a light on this poorly understood eye condition from a patient's perspective. The opinions expressed are my own.

Early issues with visual impairment - a bit of background

I am an Anglo-Burmese woman, born in the UK. My parents came to Britain in the late 50s. Burma is now known as Myanmar, but we still call it Burma.

I have always been short-sighted and had my first pair of glasses at the age of seven. There's a family legend that says that our poor vision stemmed from a life-threatening snakebite my mother had as a child in Burma. She was treated by a monk who saved her life.

My mum even wrote a story about this incident, she described being rushed from her home to the monastery, watching all the branches of the trees overhead as she was carried in great haste. The monk warned my mum that her vision would be affected in the future. Whilst it doesn't sound credible that a Burmese monk with limited medical training could have predicted my mother's poor eyesight, and there's certainly no clinical record for it, it does seem odd to me that it proved to be true – my mother started wearing glasses after a while and most of my siblings are short-sighted as well.

I am now in my 60s and have had a varied working life. These days, the main focus of my work is writing.

Onset of strabismus symptoms.

I learned to live with high myopia with the help of glasses and contact lenses. When I reached 50, I became increasingly worried that my eyesight would not last my lifetime. At almost every check-up, I would be told that my eyesight had deteriorated further. My very kind optician would do his best to reassure me, but he did acknowledge that my vision was very poor, and the rate of deterioration could not be put down to age alone. My high myopia did not affect my ability to work.

Prior to the onset of strabismus, I had suffered other issues with my sight, including a retinal tear in my right eye which presented as a small hole in my vision and thankfully healed by itself. In 2014, a visual field test showed up a symmetrical loss of peripheral vision that caused concern; my optician felt it was important to rule out a possible pituitary tumour pressing on the optic nerve. Thankfully, this proved not to be the case. I was told that the loss of peripheral vision was most likely an 'artefact of high myopia.'

IN 2015 I suddenly noticed double vision (diplopia) in my long-distance vision; in a theatre one person on a stage would look like two overlapping people. Also, when looking out for a bus in the distance, again the bus would be two overlapping images. It was alarming and annoying. I was referred to the Strabismus team at Moorfields. The treatment option of surgery was discussed, but I was reluctant to consider it at that time. I was given plain glasses with a prism that did help in a theatre but made no difference when outside looking into the distance. After a time, it seemed that there was little more to do to help me because I was not ready to consider surgery and we jointly agreed, in **2017** that I would be discharged.

In August 2018, I was on holiday in Italy, celebrating my birthday with friends. I was sitting at a computer when I noticed, with horror, that the lines on the screen were swimming, overlapping horizontally as I typed. I found myself re-reading the same line of typed text. I was also unwell with a horrible allergic skin reaction to an insect bite. I hoped that the distressing central double vision would clear once I recovered from the allergic reaction. I wanted to believe that the two were somehow linked. Sadly, this was not the case. The allergic skin reaction passed quite quickly, but the awful double-vision in my immediate central vision remained. I found it deeply depressing and hard to accept.

On my return to London, I attended an emergency eye clinic, and it was sadly confirmed that I now had strabismus-induced diplopia in my central vision. There then followed a long period of time involving multiple hospital appointments and I had to learn to live with strabismus-induced diplopia right in my central vision, as well as my long-distance vision.

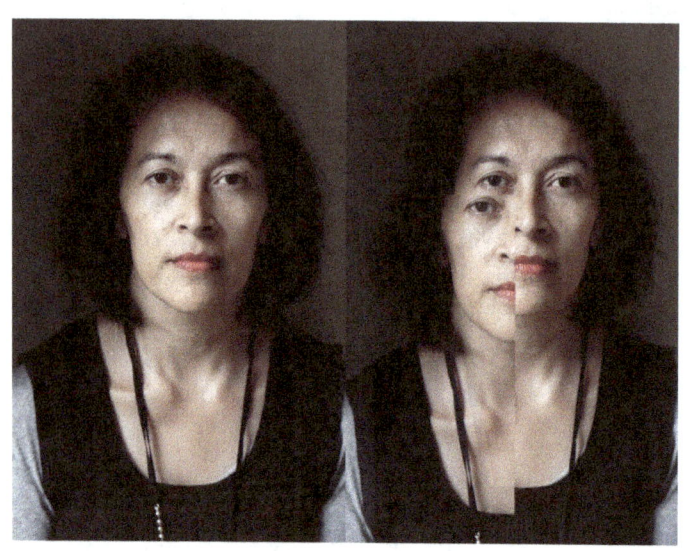

Living with the impact of strabismus

So, what is it like living with strabismus/a squint? Before I explain some of the things I suffered, I want to consider the following question, in my own, layperson's terms.

What is strabismus?

Strabismus is the medical term for a squint. it means the patient has misaligned eyes. However, the term 'a squint' is quite misleading when it comes to trying to explain what strabismus really is for a sufferer. In fact, during my research for this book, I've discovered that there's quite a linguistic muddle around the terms *strabismus* and *a squint* which I've elaborated on in the section, **Words Matter**.

So, let me return to what it was like living with strabismus.

There were many unpleasant aspects which definitely interfered with my activities of daily living. Here are some examples:

A. Increased 'clumsiness', more accidents.

Not all patients with strabismus have diplopia/double-vision, but I certainly did. When you can see two images overlapping for example, a cup you are trying to pick up, or a door handle you are trying to grasp, you will have accidents. I tripped on steps because I wasn't sure which was the real edge, versus the 'ghost' edge. I broke precious items because I've knocked them over having misjudged where they actually were. I injured my arm when I tried to go through a doorway with a very heavy door and the door fell back on my arm causing a massive bruise because I couldn't work out where the real edges of the doorway were. I learned to be extra careful as I went about. It was tiring to be so careful all the time.

I was using touch to help me sometimes, feeling my way to reassure myself that what I see is truly what is in front of me. I would use my heel when walking down steps in the underground, tapping it against the back of the step before I proceeded down to the next step. Interestingly, a young patient waiting in the same clinic told me that she was using some of the same techniques to manage.

B. Computer usage became more difficult, more tiring than it used to be.

I tried to think of ways to make things easier and I discovered that if I printed text that was on screen, it was easier to read and less likely to go double, if at all. I later discussed this with an Orthoptist who explained that the reason for this was that the contrast on a screen was less/there were fewer pixels than on the printed page. I called RNIB (Royal National Institute of Blind People) who had lots of advice, including information on adjusting my workstation. I continued to work normally but the double-vision was worse when I was tired, and I had more headaches as a consequence.

C. A 'creased' landscape

When I was outdoors, in nature, the landscape was like a photograph with a big crease down the middle. I couldn't really enjoy being outside as I used to as the view was fractured and jumbled. I love looking at nature, taking walks and visiting a beach but these activities were no longer the pleasure they once were because of the distortion in my sight.

D. Cosmetic appearance

We all want to look our best and I know that I didn't look as I used to, albeit that the misalignment of my eyes was not very obvious. Still, it made me sad. Some people with strabismus have noticeably misaligned eyes, which makes them self-conscious.

I've heard that some people don't understand the use of Botox injections for squint. Botox is more commonly known now for freezing wrinkles but the

Botox injections for squint is a medical treatment to improve the patient's vision, by stabilising the muscles. It's troubling to think that this misapprehension is leading people to underestimate the impact of strabismus and may even lead to the cutting of treatment by health commissioners.

E. Cruel jokes/ No Laughing Matter

Strabismus is not only poorly understood, but also sometimes a cause for humour. I have had people close to me make jokes that they think are funny, not meant cruelly. I don't find it funny at all, but I suppose it's because comic characters and 'fools' are often shown on TV and in films as a cross-eyed person for some reason. The 'village idiot' stereotype is often shown with misaligned eyes. I've seen examples of this on TV comedy shows quite recently. Do an internet search of 'village idiot' or 'idiot face' and see what images come up! It is not surprising that people with strabismus (a squint) are self-conscious about their appearance.

F. The human element.

I couldn't look people in the eye as I used to, it made me feel furtive, self-conscious. I would often hide behind my hair, covering one eye. It is especially upsetting in relation to looking at loved ones, for example when I am sitting in a restaurant with a double image of the person opposite. I couldn't really connect with the other person's eyes. It was so frustrating and emotionally isolating; it broke the connection between me and the other person. I would wear an eye patch sometimes because it cut out the diplopia, but, understandably, that made me self-conscious as well.

Surgery

In 2019 I transferred my care to the Royal Free Hospital which is my own local hospital. where I met Mr Jain and his wonderful team of orthoptists, nurses, registrars, and clinic staff.

Mr Jain was very patient and thorough in explaining my condition and the treatment and I finally felt able to overcome my fear and commit to surgery. As I also had cataracts in both eyes, the plan was to do my cataract surgery first. Both cataract operations were carried out in 2019.

As someone who has lived all her adult life, and much of her childhood wearing glasses and contact lenses, it felt nothing less than miraculous to be able to see without glasses or contact lenses! I cried when I took the bandage off following the cataract surgery.

Next, I had to wait for the strabismus surgery. I knew that there were risks involved, especially for high myopes like me, but I desperately longed to be rid of the double vision in my central vision.

This was booked for March 2020, and I count myself lucky that the procedure went ahead because, days later, the covid pandemic was formally declared and all non-urgent eye surgery was cancelled.

Mr Jain performed the Yokoyama procedure which involved moving some of the muscles in my right eye to ensure the normal anatomy was restored, as a day-case and everything went well.
The following day, when I woke up, I looked up at the overhead light and was so happy to see just one light – not double! When I got up and moved around everything was single again, no more double vision! Only someone who has lived with diplopia resulting from strabismus can really appreciate what a blessed relief it was to no longer have double vision.

I don't want my statement to suggest that my experience of strabismus is exactly the same for everyone else. Strabismus, in its most simple description, means the patient has misaligned eyes, a squint in everyday terms. However, as you will see from the interviews with Marilena, Anna Maria and Paul, and from the photographs created for the book, strabismus is a serious eye condition which can create several different issues. Moreover, there is a significant psychological impact as well as negative effects on activities of daily living.

It is very disappointing that this eye condition is not taken as seriously as it should be.
I fear that the underestimating of the impact of this eye condition may be leading to poorer availability of treatment and inadequate support for patients with strabismus.
This is my personal view.

I am extremely grateful for the excellent treatment and support I received from Mr Jain and his team at the Royal Free and I wish the same for all sufferers of strabismus. I am so thankful that I continue to enjoy good vision, without distortion,
without strabismus.

Diptych of Lucia illustrating diplopia caused by strabismus.

Original photograph by Francesca Cesari –
Diptych created in collaboration with Lucia Wilson

4. The Medical Perspective with Mr Saurabh Jain, consultant ophthalmologist,

Mr Jain is a Consultant Ophthalmologist and Clinical Director, Royal Free Hospital, London
Senior Personal Tutor and Honorary Associate Professor, UCL Medical School.

Hello, Saurabh, Francesca and I have been delighted to have your participation in our project, Face to Face with Strabismus, and we are very grateful to be able to interview you.

Firstly, could you start by telling us a bit about yourself and a) your work here in the UK, in general b) and, more specifically, your work on strabismus for children and adults?

I am a consultant surgeon specialising in the treatment of eye disorders in children and strabismus in children and adults. I did my initial training in London and then decided to specialise further in the treatment of disorders of eye movements.

I undertook specialised fellowships in paediatric ophthalmology and strabismus in Leicester and Manchester before commencing my consultant post at the Royal Free Hospital in 2009. In addition, I work as an honorary associate professor at UCL medical school and am affiliated with various international organisations dedicated to the study of strabismus.

My work is divided almost equally between treating adults with motility disorders and various paediatric ophthalmology conditions. It is a very fulfilling and complex job role with many challenges but also a lot of satisfaction. I also do a significant amount of teaching and training both for postgraduate doctors as well as for the medical school. I have published a textbook about simplifying strabismus diagnosis and management for more junior eye professionals to spread awareness about this condition.

Strabismus (a squint) is a complex condition, yet it seems to have a very simple description in some dictionaries i.e., *a condition in which the two eyes point in different directions.* **Could you tell us, in lay terms, more about strabismus/a squint and the different conditions that can cause it?**

Are the causes of strabismus in adults different to the causes in children and babies? Could you talk a bit about this?

I think that is quite a good description. Strabismus is a condition where the eyes are not aligned perfectly and therefore point in different directions. There are two main types of strabismus. Congenital or childhood strabismus is seen in children or young adults and is present either at birth or in the first few years of life. It tends to be primarily horizontal and measures the same in every direction of gaze. Children tend not to get double vision with strabismus as their brains are more adaptable. However, it can be associated with a lazy eye or the need for glasses which are usually treated before the eye misalignment can be corrected. No one really knows why some children develop strabismus, but we know that prematurity and a family history of strabismus make it more likely. In contrast, adults tend to present with acquired strabismus, which is usually following a discrete event such as trauma or stroke or alternatively associated with age or high refractive disorders like myopia etc. This kind of strabismus tends to be usually associated with double vision and therefore is treated differently with glasses, toxin, or surgery.

Orthoptists play a key role in the treatment of strabismus, but few people know about their work, could you talk to us about the role of orthoptists?

Orthoptists are absolutely crucial to the assessment of strabismus. They tend to be the first professionals that see strabismus patients in eye clinics and carry out measurement of the deviation of the eyes as well as an assessment of the motility of the eyes. They carry out eye tests in children, that can't always be easily done in the community, to help treat disorders like lazy eyes and also support the eye clinics in the treatment of other conditions such as glaucoma and macular degeneration.

Do you think that strabismus patients in the UK are well supported with good access to treatment?

The secondary care for strabismus, i.e., in the hospital setting is quite good in my opinion and most eye departments will have orthoptists and a surgeon dedicated to paediatric ophthalmology and strabismus. However, the referral routes into hospital are not always easy and in a number of cases people are told that 'nothing can be done' for their strabismus which delays the referral.

Is the treatment of strabismus developing? Is there ongoing research?

Like everything we are learning more and more about strabismus every day. We know that with correct conservative management for example, the number of patients that need surgical correction can be much reduced and we are operating on fewer patients as a result. We also have newer microsurgical techniques that enable patients to achieve faster recovery with minimal scarring and I often lecture and write about these. Lastly, non-surgical methods of correction of strabismus such as botulinum toxin (or botox) are used much more commonly than they used to be.

Before I had strabismus I had never heard of the term, although I had heard of a squint. Why is so little known about strabismus?

Squint is a term that is used very commonly but it means different things to different people. Some people use it to mean 'screwing the eyes up" while others use it synonymously with strabismus which means the eyes are pointing in different directions and to my mind the latter is the preferred term as there is no ambiguity in the meaning.

Now that you have had time to review the photography and the interviews with Marilena and Anna Maria (in Italy) and Paul (who is one of your own patients as well) along with my own

statement about my experience with strabismus, could you share your observations, please? Have the interviews thrown up any ideas/points that you would like to highlight?

I think it's very interesting that the same concepts come up again and again. It is the continuous presence of a disfiguring condition that on one hand is not acknowledged as a serious problem by the world at large but on the other has a profound effect on social interactions and ultimately self-image. It is also striking to hear the accounts of those who have had surgery and noticed it can produce a significant improvement.

I am reminded of a patient mine with strabismus that was completely corrected after surgery. She was very emotional after the procedure as she described to me how the strabismus had been affecting her life. In spite of it being a small deviation, it led to constant double vision which hampered almost all aspects of her life. She remembered seeing her friends waving to her from across the room at a restaurant, but getting to them was almost impossible for her as all she could see was a maze of tables and chairs to navigate through. So, her strabismus was profoundly disabling to her in spite of being practically invisible to others. This double vision completely disappeared after her surgery.

And looking specifically at the photography do you have any comments you would like to share with us? Of course, you will recall that the diptych that I created with Francesca's original photography came about out of my own frustration with diplopia and its impact, perhaps you could comment on that first of all, thinking back to when you first saw it?

I think the photographs are very striking as they depict how the patients perceive their own self and the world around them, and I think that's something that we as medical professionals don't maybe pay as much attention to as we should.

The diptych for example beautifully illustrates the impact of the world seen as similar overlapping images. I was also very taken by the pictures of the

Italian patient covering her eyes as if wanting not to be seen. I see this all the time as people try to cover their 'deformity' by either refusing to meet my gaze during consultation or growing their hair in such a way that it covers one eye. One can only imagine the effect of this on their self confidence in our image obsessed world.

It is also really heart breaking to read these accounts and realise that it has taken a long time for people to get access to the treatment that they needed to make the most of their potential.

As a former sufferer of strabismus, I think strabismus is not well understood by the general public. I also think it's often dismissed as a minor condition. Strabismus patients don't get much sympathy in my experience. What do you think about that? Have other patients expressed this view?

I agree and I speak a bit about that above. It is dismissed as a cosmetic problem by insurance companies and even by medical professionals at times and I spend a lot of time explaining to people that it is not cosmetic as we are not enhancing anything but merely restoring things to how they should be. There is also a mistaken assumption that strabismus is linked to poor intelligence as you have alluded to in your 'village idiot' comments.

In your role as an educator training new doctors in ophthalmology, are you excited/confident about the future care of strabismus patients?
Are there new treatment options or exciting developments on the horizon? If so, please tell us more.

As I said, I spend lot of my time teaching and training, and we are facing a real crisis in the recruitment of specialists within paediatric ophthalmology and strabismus. It is seen as a difficult specialty to train in, with complex patients and often not much fame or remuneration as compared to say cataract or refractive surgery specialists. I am trying to change the perception of residents by showing them the varied presentations of strabismus and the impact that the surgery can have on people's lives and sense of self-worth.

I am the Education officer for BIPOSA which is the British and Irish Paediatric Ophthalmology and Strabismus Association. This is a fantastic organisation that seeks to promote the awareness of eye conditions among children and adults with strabismus as well as treatment options available to them. I am very honoured to be organising the annual meeting of the organisation in London in autumn this year (2023).

You are the author of *Simplifying Strabismus* – could you tell us a bit more about your book?

This is a book I wrote a few years ago, aimed at residents in Ophthalmology to simplify the study of strabismus by presenting cases and management options in an easy to read, logical format along with lots of clinical videos and diagrams. I am very fortunate in that the book has been received with a lot of enthusiasm across the world and has now been commissioned for a second edition by Springer.

5. The Medical Perspective with strabismologist, Dr. Giovanni Battista Marcon, in Italy

Dr Marcon is also the founder and director of the Strabismus and Diplopia Centre in Bassano del Grappa.

Hello, Giovanni, Francesca and I have been delighted to have your participation in our project, Face to Face with Strabismus, and we are very grateful to be able to interview you
Firstly, could you start by telling us a bit about yourself and a) your work in Italy, in general and b) more specifically, your work on strabismus, for children and adults?

My name is Giovanni Battista Marcon, I am an Italian ophthalmologist, 62 years old. I specialized in ophthalmology when I was 29 years old and had gone through all the steps of a hospital career: from resident to head of the ophthalmological department at Gorizia-Monfalcone Public Hospital.

I am mainly an eye surgeon. In my career I've performed around 18,000 cataract surgeries and also hundreds of glaucoma, retina and keratoplasty operations and thousands of strabismus surgeries.

I have been fascinated by strabismus and strabismus surgery since I was a young ophthalmologist but couldn't dedicate myself totally to this field because of the amount of routine surgery in the hospital.

When I was 49 years old, I decided to leave the hospital (and my position as head of ophthalmology) and to dedicate myself full-time to strabismus and strabismus surgery. There were many reasons that drove me to take this important decision but two of the most significant are:

a) very few ophthalmologists in Italy dedicate their time to the cure of strabismus.

b) despite this, the satisfaction that the surgeon and the patient derive from a well-conducted strabismus treatment is enormous.

In 2009, I left the hospital and founded the Diplopia and Strabismus Centre in Bassano del Grappa, the city where I live.

Since then, I have dedicated all my time to curing strabismus in children and adults.

Strabismus is a complex condition, yet it seems to have a very simple description i.e., to have misaligned eyes. In layman's terms, could you tell us more about strabismus and the different conditions that can cause it? For example, do you see many patients with myopia who go on to develop strabismus? Can you talk about diplopia and strabismus? Do all patients with strabismus have diplopia?

Strabismus is basically a misalignment of the two eyes; they are no longer straight and hence they don't fix on the same target.

There are many causes of Strabismus. It may be congenital or linked to a particular refractive error (hyperopia or myopia), it may be caused by a damage to one or more of the three oculomotor nerves that innervates extraocular muscles, it may be caused by systemic diseases: thyroid disease, Parkinson disease. It may be iatrogenic strabismus.

What is important to understand, is that whatever the cause is, in relation to the age of onset (mainly children or adults) it causes different adaptation or symptoms. During childhood (from 0 to 6 years old) strabismus will not cause diplopia (with some exceptions) because the brain adapts to this condition and suppresses the image of the deviated eye. This prevents diplopia appearing but may cause amblyopia and therefore loss of vision.

During adulthood the onset of a strabismus causes "confusion" and "diplopia " no matter the causes. The patient will be invariably disturbed and will have a reduction in quality of life.

High myopia is a frequent cause of strabismus in adulthood. Myopia is present since adolescence, but strabismus appears, in these patients, in their 40s or 50s. It may be with acute onset or progressive onset. In this case, the patient tries, unconsciously to adapt to diplopia and confusion and misunderstands symptoms for a long time.

This may be a cause of delay in the diagnosis with patients trying to change glasses to improve their vision.

Strabismus may also occur in low myopia and in younger patients.

Do you see more female patients than male patients? Or is there no obvious difference?

No, the incidence of strabismus is approximately the same in both sexes.

Orthoptists play a key role in the treatment of strabismus, but few people know about their work, could you talk to us about the role of orthoptists?

Yes, the orthoptist is important in the diagnosis and follow-up of strabismus.

Unfortunately, in my country, few ophthalmologists give proper attention to strabismus and therefore they don't operate on strabismus patients.

Hence most orthoptists are used differently in hospitals. They perform visual fields, OCT, or other practical examinations to support the ophthalmologist's work but don't specifically take care of strabismus patients. When an orthoptist works together with a strabismologist (an ophthalmologist specializing in strabismus) it creates the best team for diagnosing and treating strabismus.

Do you think that strabismus patients in Italy are well supported with good access to treatment?

No. Unfortunately strabismus patients, in particular adults, are not well supported in Italy, but this is also the case, with some differences, in other countries.

There are many reasons for this, at least in Italy. First of all, strabismology is a complex ophthalmological sub-specialty where you need to study a lot. It may be very difficult, for a young ophthalmologist, to understand, at the beginning, how to treat or operate on a strabismus patient, particularly an adult.

Secondly, ophthalmology is a very technical medical specialty full of devices and equipment, for example lasers (excimer, YAG, Argon, femtoseconds lasers), phacoemulsifiers, vitrectomy, endo lights etc, etc. The opportunity to use these machines attracts young ophthalmologists, but this is not the case in strabismology.

When I was a young ophthalmologist I was attracted as well by this world so I can understand them, but this fact leaves strabismology (at least in Italy) neglected.

Is the treatment of strabismus developing? Is there ongoing research?

Yes. There is a lot of research going on that is basically refining the techniques and knowledge developed in the 70's and 80's but also discover new strabismus and new etiopathogenesis. From this point of view the use of imaging in strabismology, namely MRI, in the last 15 years has been fundamental. Through MRI we now are able to demonstrate, for instance, the ageing of extraocular muscles, we can measure muscle contraction and paths. For me the combination of the clinical data and the anatomical data provided by MRI gives the patient the maximum chance to understand well his/her strabismus and hence we can design the best surgical strategy.

Before I had strabismus I had never heard of the term, although I had heard of a squint. Why is so little known about strabismus? And is this part of the reason why it's not taken seriously by some people?

In my opinion, at least in my country, strabismus has been considered for a long time an "aesthetic" problem. It is commonly thought that an aesthetic problem is not serious and doesn't deserve much attention. Now we definitely know that this is not

true, and that strabismus causes a lot of problems for patients, but this message is not completely and fully
understood by the general public, and even by some ophthalmologists.

As you know, I am writing a section called Words Matter where I have made some research into the usage of the phrase 'a squint' versus the medical name 'strabismus'. You confirmed that, in Italian, there is only one word for strabismus *strabismo,* and that the Italian translation for a squint is also *strabismo.*

Yes I can confirm that.

I have a theory that these two words in English are causing some linguistic confusion which might actually be having an impact on the way patients are treated – what are your thoughts on that? Does the use of two expressions (in English) for strabismus cause complications for Italian

specialists as well? You informed me that all international strabismus conferences are conducted in English. We'd be grateful for your comments on this point.

Yes, all International Meetings about strabismus are conducted in English. This may be a problem because orthoptists or ophthalmologists that don't speak or understand English may choose not to participate. There are, of course, National Strabismus Meetings in all countries but the advantage, in International Meetings, is that you have all Opinion Leaders of each country in one Meeting and the update is more comprehensive and higher level.

For example, E.S.A. (European Strabismological Association) of which I am Secretary, organises a Meeting in Europe every year.

This Meeting is attended, on average, by only 5-10 Italians (Ophthalmologists and Orthoptists) mainly because of language problems and high expenses.

I think the fact that strabismus generally doesn't attract a lot of funding is one reason why this condition is less well-known and therefore poorly supported. Sadly, most hospitals in Italy will not fund the attendance of their orthoptists and doctors at international strabismus conferences which further hampers the sharing of knowledge in relation to strabismus.

Now that you have had time to review the photography of and the interviews with Marilena and Anna Maria, two of your own patients, and Paul (UK patient), along with my own statement about my experience with strabismus, could you comment on them, please?

Anna Maria and Marilena are two typical examples of Italian adult strabismus patients. They suffered a lot because of their condition in the past (strabismus) and wanted to improve but they didn't find an answer. They were told for years that "the condition cannot be treated or even improved," that their strabismus was not curable.

Huge is the wonder, the surprise, and the joy when they find a surgeon that tells them the truth: strabismus is treatable, and surgery gives excellent results.

I think their comments and also their photographs express this inner happiness: Marilena because she has finally improved her strabismus and Anna Maria because she is waiting for her surgery.

As a former sufferer of strabismus, I feel that strabismus is not well understood and subsequently dismissed as a minor condition. Strabismus patients don't get much sympathy in my experience. What do you think about that? Have you observed this reaction in your own patients?

Yes, of course. Before being a strabismologist and hence operating only on strabismus, I have been a" general" ophthalmic surgeon. I have performed around 18,000 cataract surgeries in my career, hundreds of glaucoma surgeries, and retinal detachment surgeries and also keratoplastic surgeries (corneal transplantation).

I can assure you that the satisfaction, the happiness, and the joy of a well-operated strabismus patient is unique. We, as human beings, are made to use our eyes together and when you regain binocular vision this gives you eye health and inner and outer well-being that is not comparable with other eye surgeries.

Do you think that strabismus is well understood in the medical community in Italy, generally? When we spoke online, you talked about a lack of awareness at the primary care/GP level – could you say more about that, please?

As I said before, strabismus is not well understood in the medical community (GPs but also Ophthalmologists). There is a general lack of awareness about the importance of correcting this condition. This is a pity because a lot of patients could be treated, improving their quality of life, and, instead, they are left with their strabismus.

Are you excited/confident about the future care of strabismus patients in Italy?

I am confident because of the huge possibilities we have now to diagnose and treat strabismus particularly in adults. At the same time, I am disillusioned because, in my country, I see very few young ophthalmologists that want to become strabismologists.

No Joke
- Lucia Wilson

Laughter is often described as the best medicine. I agree, laughing eases tension and fills us with delight. I love a good joke and I like to include humour in my stories for children and adults. It's well known that there are all sorts of positive benefits – social, physical, and mental - from shared laughter.

But what if you are the butt of the joke? What if some aspect of your physical appearance, something entirely beyond your control is the root of someone else's joke?

I suffered with strabismus for several years, and during that time, I became aware of the cruel mocking of people with misaligned eyes. On one occasion I was accused of having a 'sense of humour failure' when I felt hurt and didn't laugh at a joke about my strabismus. Other strabismus sufferers have had similar experiences.

I have seen recent TV shows (as recent as 2022) – from the UK and the USA – where a character has been ridiculed for their misaligned eyes. In one UK show, a comedian deliberately made his eyes go out of alignment in order to represent someone who was of low intelligence.

In one American comedy drama, a woman was selecting a potential date for her friend from an online dating site; she rejected one man that she called 'the squinty guy' (he had misaligned eyes) along with all the other men she said were unattractive and not good enough to date her friend.

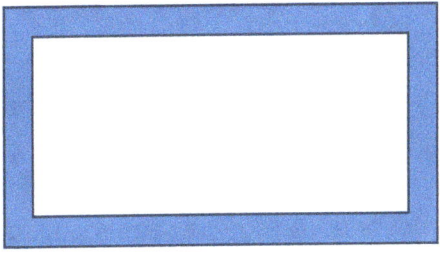

Let me set you an exercise if I may. Think about the empty box above and search the internet for a photograph or illustration related to 'an idiot' 'village idiot' 'fool' 'stupid person' to place into that box.

You will find various images online that show a person with misaligned eyes. You will also find stock libraries who provide such photographs and illustrations today. There are also numerous 'silly face' emojis that use misaligned eyes as a key component of the illustration. This shows that the hurtful and totally erroneous link between low intelligence/silliness and misaligned eyes is seen as acceptable, even today.

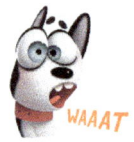

How has this association evolved? Why does such a correlation persist? I'm not qualified to address this question, so I don't propose to answer it here, but I do want to provoke some discussion of this point. I think it's cruel and unkind to use misaligned eyes to illustrate low intelligence. I think it's harmful to children and adults with strabismus.

Many patients with strabismus are already self-conscious about their eyes, they'll often hide behind their hair or cover their eyes with a hand or drop their head low to avoid meeting someone else's eyes. It really adds insult to injury to find that a visual impairment beyond your control is a point of mockery and ridicule. It's a further indication of the negative impact of having strabismus and it's no laughing matter.

7. The Psychological Element with Dr Silvia Riva, psychologist and lecturer, London

Dr Silvia Riva is an Associate Professor of Psychology at St Mary's University, London, and a practicing HCPC clinical psychologist at DottoreLondon.

Hello Silvia, thank you so much for your work and support with our project.
As an Italian national working in the UK, you have experience of both countries which means you not only bring your psychological expertise to our project, but also with lived experience of both countries and patients in both countries and we are very grateful for your involvement.

Can we begin by asking you to tell us a bit about you and your work?

Hello, I am Silvia, and I am an associate professor of psychology at St Mary's University. I also do clinical activities with patients in London. A major area of research and work with patients is health-related quality of life. The HRQOL is a multidimensional construct that encompasses at least three broad domains - physical, psychological, and social functioning - that may be affected by one's illness or treatment. HRQOL is usually measured in chronic conditions and is often adversely affected. Through my career, I have explored this topic in a variety of chronic conditions and in cancer survivors.

Now that you have had time to read the patient interviews – two patients from Italy and two from the UK, including my own statement (Lucia) are there any observations about living with strabismus that you would like to share?

The stories of these patients were profound and full of courage. As I observed their daily lives, their work, their relationships with others, and their relationship with the mirror, I was struck by their incredible ability to adapt strabismus to their everyday lives. While strabismus is certainly a painful aspect of their lives, their adaptation, or psychologically, their coping, shows an incredible ability to deal with the inner suffering caused by feeling different.

I was very impressed with all the strength of these stories, which, on a psychological level, demonstrate a great deal of resilience. A person who is resilient is someone who is capable of successfully adapting to difficult or challenging life experiences, especially through mental, emotional, and behavioral flexibility and adjustment to external and internal pressures. We can all learn from these stories.

Looking at the photographs, can you comment on these?

The eyes serve as communicative elements of our bodies with which we interact. There is much information conveyed by these eyes; they are eyes that tell a story, not always an easy or painless one. However, they also convey very positive aspects. As well as expressing courage and depth, they also convey a sense of strength.

The misalignment of a strabismus patient's eyes can sometimes be very obvious to other people and the reactions of other people can impact the strabismus patient's self-esteem in relation to their self-image, could you talk more about that? Could you consider how this might impact children, who also suffer with strabismus?

It has been reported that people with strabismus suffer from low self-esteem because they often struggle with interpersonal relationships and social anxiety. This is primarily due to the fact that these individuals find it difficult to integrate strabismus with their body image and face image, and they feel that
they are very different from others. This situation can be very hard when you are a child. During the early years of childhood (between pre-school and primary school), we all develop our social identity, which is partly determined by our inner characteristics and personality factors, but also by our interactions with other children. When we believe we are significantly different from others, we tend to stay very distant from them. Feeling different makes people feel distant from others. Psychologically, this behaviour might lead to difficulty in maintaining social

relationships and might lead to a fear of social situations or an avoidance of them. The psychological development of children with strabismus should be supported by a psychologist. However, it is also important to operate at the community level and educate other children and other individuals regarding the condition of these children and how we can help them.

Sometimes other people are quite cruel towards strabismus patients, mocking their misaligned eyes. I have seen several recent examples of TV comedy shows referring to people with a noticeable squint/strabismus in a negative, rejecting way (a sign of ugliness and/or even stupidity) can you discuss what kind of impact this might have on an adult? Can you also comment on the impact this might have on a child with strabismus?

We all experience superficiality and vanity for different reasons. Social media and television are often responsible for increasing the level of superficiality. Our reliance upon others' superficiality can be detrimental to us; people rely heavily on what others say as part of the process of developing their identity. It is important, however, not to "absorb" everything we hear. We don't have the power to eliminate superficiality, but, with our minds, we have the power to always do two important things: 1) Do not generalise negative remarks about oneself; recognise that people are not all fools and that there are many non-superficial people who can enrich our life, 2) Don't focus on everything, but rather on something important and meaningful to our lives.

For some strabismus patients, looking into the eyes of another person can be difficult. For me, personally, I found it quite isolating. Given that looking into the eyes of other people is such a fundamental part of human relationships, especially with loved ones, what do you think of the impact of this on people with strabismus?

It is evident from these stories that this difficulty causes a great deal of suffering. Psychologically, suffering is characterised by avoidance, isolation, and pain. For us to be able to offer appropriate assistance, we should always listen to suffering and learn from these stories. I have found these stories to be very inspirational.

And can we also discuss a theme that we considered when we first met you, and that is the issue of perfectionism in terms of physical appearance. We would be grateful to hear your opinion of this not only in terms of strabismus but for patients with other visible physical impairments and disabilities.

Whether it is in terms of physical appearance or other aspects of one's professional or private life, perfectionism has many shades. Mass media and a continuous push to popularize perfect bodies and faces certainly contribute to physical perfectionism. On a psychological level, perfectionism is rooted in a universal human weakness known as the "illusion of control": the illusion of control over time, age, or appearance. Realistically, we have no such control, and our lives flow independently of one another.

My personal opinion is that we would be better served by not paying attention to messages of perfectionism. It is important that we focus on our own goals and the values that inspire us to give our lives a realistic direction.

And finally, can you offer some general advice for

a) an adult struggling with the impact of strabismus
b) a parent caring for a child with strabismus

In both cases, I believe it is vital to have psychological support that assists us in overcoming our fears and emotions as well as boosting our self-esteem in order to be able to live a peaceful life.

In my opinion, it is very important to start a path alongside medical treatments; medicine and psychology are not separate disciplines, so they must work together in order to provide adequate support to patients.

8. The Photographic Perspective
with Francesca Cesari

Francesca, could you begin by talking a bit about yourself and your work as a photographer?

My name is Francesca Cesari and I'm a freelance photographer based in Bologna, Italy.
I have a Master's Degree in Contemporary Art History and while I was studying at the University of Bologna I started my activity as a self-taught photographer. I then perfected my skills at the London College of Printing, where I attended a one-year training course in Professional Photographic Practice.

Along with commercial assignments and teaching photography I mainly work with long-term personal projects, where the main element of my visual language is portraiture. Most of all I focus on people, exploring relationships, adolescence and women's issues and I'm particularly interested in some of the key phases of human lives, when transformation and change are particularly evident.

I love to portray people in their environment, I like the atmosphere that lived places give to a scene and the way people move inside their natural space - that's why I almost always work on location with natural light.

You and I are the co-creators of the Face to Face project, from which the book, Face to Face with Strabismus has evolved and you and I have worked closely together on it from its inception. However, I'd like to ask you, as the photographer, about your thoughts regarding your photographic work for Face to Face with Strabismus.

Can you begin by talking about how this project came about and why it stimulated your interest as a photographer?

As creative people, you and I have often discussed working together on a project in our respective roles of photographer and writer. Strangely, it was the onset of your strabismus that led us to the creation of the wider project of Face to Face and Face to Face with Strabismus grew out of that. A photograph that I took of you in 2014 formed the basis of a diptych that was pivotal to this.

I recall that you contacted me because you wanted to use my original photograph to help to illustrate how you saw yourself in the mirror. You talked about how

frustrating it was to have diplopia and how other people didn't understand how debilitating it was. You explained that your diplopia (caused by the strabismus) meant that your reflection was severely distorted. You printed that portrait and with a *collage* you placed my original photograph of you (unaltered) next to the distorted image.

Mr Saurabh Jain, your consultant ophthalmologist, shared this image via social media as an illustration of what strabismus patients with diplopia suffer. I then worked on this diptych to create a further enhanced form of the diptych which is the version of this compelling image today.

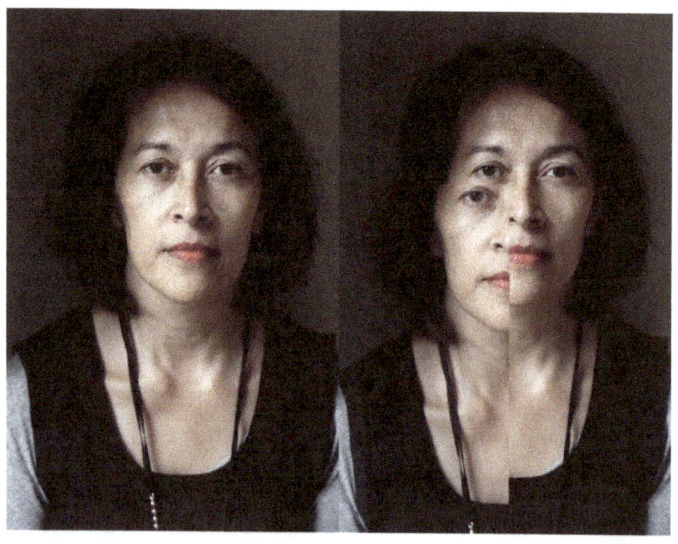

We talked a lot about that diptych and about the psychological implications that a person with visual impairment could have because of a distorted vision. The concept of the project *Face to Face* was born and we started to develop the idea of working on different forms of visual impairments (both through photography and writing), having in mind the production of a book and an exhibition.

As a photographer I was fascinated by the chance of working with the concept of distorted vision connected to portraiture, the idea of exploring such a delicate and personal topic as self-perception, especially for people affected with eye conditions, was a great opportunity to examine in depth the consideration of self-image.

I'd like to add that, by digitally manipulating the portrait I took of you in order to show your double vision, I definitely realised up close how much you must have suffered in the acute phase of your strabismus. With that kind of distorted vision any daily task and movement could be extremely challenging or even dangerous, with the consequence of feeling
unstable and insecure, an insidious and disabling problem, all the more so because it's not visible to others.

Talking about my distorted reflection, led us to an interesting discussion about self-image and mirrors,

including self-image and visual impairment. Can you share some of your thoughts about that?

I think that the mirror has always been an incredibly powerful element, a sort of magical object that gives back our appearance in a mixture of objectivity (the physical reality of our reflected image) and subjectivity (the way we look at ourselves through our eyes). Mirrors give us an idea of what the others see when they look at us, yet they equally reflect what we want (or we prefer) to see: we could turn, choose our favourite side, smile, wink, make a seductive gaze, a reliable expression, a funny face; we can rehearse different versions of ourselves and stay with the ones we are more in tune with.

It's more difficult to look at ourselves in the mirror with a perfectly neutral expression, because, in my opinion, we tend to look for perfectionism or, at least, for the best version of ourselves, a look that is often

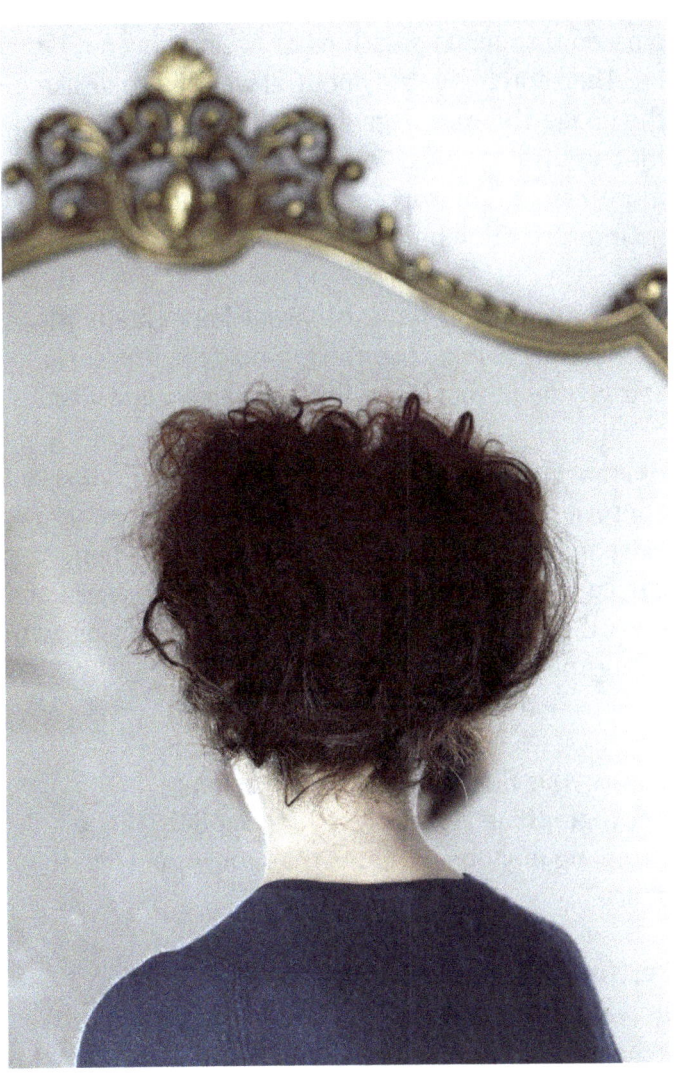

created through expressions or posing - even if just a bit. Therefore, if we stay neutral we tend to dislike the image the mirror gives back to us, but is exactly that neutral, "naked" expression that interests me more as a photographer, just because there's no interpretation but a sheer human presence.

I believe that the issue of visual impairment fits in this already complex context, amplifying the sense of estrangement that the reflected image could give.

Hearing your explanation of living with diplopia, I can appreciate that this must have been alienating and extremely hard to cope with, especially when your eye condition is not visible to the external world and the others can't guess the difficulties of living with strabismus.

This is your first experience, I believe, of photographing visually impaired models; did it throw up any observations that you would like to share?

Yes, this is my first time working with visually impaired sitters.
When I photograph people I usually try to have a very respectful approach, I'm aware that it takes a good

deal of courage to sit in front of the camera, indeed taking a portrait is an intimate exchange between people.

My experience with Marilena and Anna Maria was very positive and intense. I didn't act differently from other sessions, yet I felt I had to be particularly delicate, because the eyes -in addition of being usually the key focus of the portraits - were also a part of their body that was particularly vulnerable for my models, therefore I tried to follow their way of sitting or moving without directing too much the shoot. I asked them to be as neutral as possible and they responded really well, in a very honest and generous way.

As a photographer with a special interest in portraiture, has the experience of working on our project added to your own knowledge (from a photographic and artistic perspective?)

Working on this project has allowed me to investigate deeper the concept of portraiture, not only in its photographic meaning but in its perceptive, existential aspect.

Looking at oneself in the mirror is already a way of taking a portrait, people with visual impairment have a different approach to self-image, because the means with which they're able to see is the very sense that has something wrong with it, so the whole process of looking at oneself is strongly conditioned by it. It's a game of Chinese boxes where it's easy to get lost, so I've learned to be even more sensitive and respectful when approaching my sitters.

As you recall, we had a lively discussion about the role of the photographer and my desire, especially as a former patient with strabismus, to try and make the portrait give the impression that the sitter was alone with themself, perhaps looking at themselves in a mirror. Can you talk about that?

As I mentioned earlier, in my opinion, being alone in front of a mirror can be one of the most intimate moments a person can experience. We are always in a close relation with ourselves, even when we are with other people in our minds we constantly talk to ourselves, and the mirror gives us the chance to stop for a second and put a face to our imaginary selves.

It is a moment of acknowledgement and (hopefully) acceptance, an opportunity of experiencing the *here and now* of ourselves. When we talked about trying to replicate that situation in the photographs we wanted to reach that intensity, a moment of focus and simple truth without distraction.

Can I ask you about your own approach to beauty? This is quite a personal question, but when you place your eye behind the camera, do you begin to see the human face as an object? Is it necessary to get the best photograph?

I don't want to sound too obvious, but for me beauty is not at all a concept limited to a definite aesthetic canon or to the mere physical aspect.
Beauty (male and female) is the precious connection with the person I have in front of me, those minutes of epiphany when a silent dialogue takes place between the photographer and the sitter, when we both are honest and open enough to let the other person establish a sincere and intense, yet transitory, communication.

Beauty is the visible potential in a person's gaze and body, it is also the strong presence of a human being who is self-aware of his limits. Beauty is the fullness of the people free to express their feelings, but it's also where there is a person who is fighting to find his way in the world.

In the end I believe beauty is very much related to the concept of being honest and true to oneself.

Can you talk about portraiture and natural light? You were very keen to use this for all the portraits. Please talk more about the human face and natural light, what's appealing about it?

Natural light is the natural condition which we usually live in, it is also the most common situation I find when I observe people and I love to replicate that atmosphere in the photographs I take.

I find natural light the best way to render people in their genuine dimension, in that element they're surrounded by it, and they relate to it when they look at the space where they live. It's not necessarily a matter of sticking to realism -I'm not a strictly documentary photographer- but a way of conveying the whole atmosphere of the scene where the sitter is placed, included the light condition.

In my work I often use reflectors to amplify or channel natural light, therefore I actually make changes to the setting I find in front of me, yet that transformation still plays with already existent elements, without interfering too much with the visual objectivity. I love to play with natural light to celebrate the subject even more, exploring ways that sometimes reveal different perspectives of the sitter which are unknown even to the subject himself.

9. Words Matter
- Lucia Wilson

You say a squint – I say strabismus.

Strabismus is the medical term for a squint. it means the patient has misaligned eyes. In fact, during my research for this book, I've discovered that there's quite a linguistic muddle around the terms *strabismus* and *a squint* which I think needs addressing.

The views I am expressing here are my own.

During the creation of our book, I have read a lot of articles and done a lot of research related to strabismus/a squint and discussed all of this with Francesca Cesari, the co-editor of this book, as well as its photographer. These discussions have helped me to clarify my own thoughts related to strabismus/a squint.

Most people who have no experience of strabismus (I mean speakers of English/with English as a first language) probably don't know the term unless they work in a medical setting or until they become a strabismus patient themselves.

Most patients with strabismus (English speakers) may not even use the term strabismus, they are more likely to call it a squint. Even though the medical term is strabismus, it's quite common to see the term a squint in NHS information handouts, in GP practices, on medical websites, in the media and so on.

I think this linguistic muddle is not helpful to patients and, indirectly, could even be hampering patient care. Why do I say that?

In everyday spoken English particularly, a squint can get mixed-up with *to squint* (to take a quick glance at something/to screw up your eyes to peer at something)

i.e., someone might say 'take a squint at... ' or 'if you squint your eyes, you can just about see..... '.

In some non-medical dictionaries, it will also give the definition 'to have misaligned eyes' but not as the primary meaning..

If I look in an Italian (non-medical dictionary) for the translation of the word a squint, I am given the word strabismo. If I look in the same Italian dictionary for the translation of the word strabismus, I am given the same word strabismo.

In fact, Dr Giovanni Battista Marcon (one of our consultants for this book) has confirmed that there is only one word for strabismus in Italian and there is no alternative word for a squint, Italian ophthalmologists use the same word for strabismus and for a squint. So, the linguistic muddle is in English only.

However, given that most international conferences about strabismus are conducted in English, as Dr Marcon informed me, it's fair to assume that the linguistic muddle continues to be a factor. It's unhelpful, at least, surely?

This mix-up in English goes further than non-medical dictionaries; I have looked at several medical dictionaries and found confusing cross-referencing between the terms a squint and strabismus. Sometimes, I have seen most of the medical details under the reference for a squint with no mention of strabismus. I have also seen some publications with no cross-reference to the term strabismus. I think it would be helpful if all the medical information were under the term strabismus.

As a patient, I found this very confusing and for a long time did not fully connect the two terms; I think this linguistic muddle is not helpful to patients.

I should say here that I am not blaming anyone for this linguistic muddle, I believe it has evolved over a very long time; language is a living entity after all.

In the UK, patients with strabismus are advised that they must alert the DVLA (the Driver and Vehicle Licensing Agency), at least that was what I was advised when I was first diagnosed with strabismus in 2016, making strabismus a notifiable health condition.

As part of our research for our book, I found the following information on the DVLA site:

"You'll need to tell DVLA if you have any of the following (even if the condition is only in one eye)

(This is an extract from the full list before the latest updates)

- *Squint (with double vision)*
- *Stargadts (juvenile macular degeneration)*
- *Strabismus (with double vision)*
- *Toxoplasma retinitis (toxoplasmosis)*
- *Visual field defects*

As you can see, at that time the DVLA listed squint and strabismus as *two* separate conditions. I suspect this happened because of the ongoing

linguistic muddle between 'squint' and 'strabismus'. I would like to make it clear that this information is no longer listed on the DVLA website, it appears that the DVLA has updated its pages regarding notifiable eye conditions in the intervening time.

However, whilst the DVLA has taken both references off their list and updated their site, it was confusing to note that the DVLA listed a squint and strabismus as two separate eye conditions and not one and the same. I don't wish to criticise the DVLA for this, but I do think it is a further illustration of the linguistic muddle around strabismus and a squint.

Is there a solution? I would like to suggest several actions:

1. That, in future, there is a concerted effort to highlight the term strabismus and lessen the usage of the term a squint when referring to misaligned eyes in any medical setting. I think opticians should be included in this.

2. I would suggest that all hospital information documents (NHS and private), online information pages are amended at the earliest

3. practical opportunity, and that all new/future publications should, at least ensure that strabismus and squint sit together with the emphasis on strabismus.
4. I would suggest that all medical dictionaries publishers should, at their next update, consider emphasising the term strabismus and put all the medical information under the term strabismus (and reduce the reference to a squint to describe it as an informal term).

The second reason I think the usage of the term a squint should be lessened is because the everyday usage of a squint trivialises the eye condition, especially because it gets mixed up with other meanings and other related words. Having strabismus/misaligned eyes isn't trivial – it should not be ignored, whether in children or adults. It's important to consult a specialist to discover the root cause and consider treatment.

There's a further reason for using the term strabismus over a squint which is that there are other meanings and other words associated with a squint that cause further confusion.

Squint can be used, informally, as an adjective to suggest an object that is not straight.

In Glasgow there is a bridge called the Clyde Arc, but locals have named it, affectionately, the Squinty Bridge because of its unusual angle. It's seen as acceptable to call the bridge the Squinty Bridge.

However, referring back to my example of the American TV show where one of the characters rejected 'the squinty guy' this is also seen to be an acceptable use of language in relation to a man with strabismus; I don't think it is. Would anyone want to hear their child with strabismus referred to as 'the squinty child'?

I am straying into the psychosocial impact of having strabismus and that is significant also. There is plenty of research around the psychosocial impact of having misaligned eyes and even in our small sample of patients (myself included) we can see evidence of this. You can read more about the psychosocial impact of having strabismus in our interview with psychologist and lecturer, Dr Silvia Riva and in the next section, *No Joke*.

So, in summary, I would like to see some ambitious (but achievable) aims taken up by all the English speaking, related professionals who deal with strabismus and eyecare in general and join me on my campaign to call strabismus by one name only in any English language setting. Let's stop calling it a squint! Yes, this is extremely ambitious, but language is a living organism. Language changes all the time and stopping the use of a squint when referring to strabismus would be a change for the better, better for strabismus patients of all ages.

10. Conclusion

At the start of this book, Francesca and I, together with the generous support and input of Mr Jain, Dr Marcon and Dr Riva, set out with one shared aim: to raise the profile of strabismus.

Through our small sample of patients who kindly provided their time, we have learnt a great deal. Having had strabismus myself, I thought I knew a lot about the condition already, but I was surprised and shocked by what we discovered. Strabismus is simple in its description, yet much more complex in reality.

With the compelling commentary from Dottore Marcon and Mr Jain, we have realised that there are clear reasons behind the lack of support for strabismus sufferers both at the primary care level and within the hospital setting, both in the UK and in Italy.

Action Point: *raise the profile of strabismus at the earliest teaching level, ensure all junior ophthalmologists are educated about strabismus.*

Some strabismus sufferers are being told, incorrectly, that there is no cure, no treatment. Why is this happening? This needs to be addressed.

Action Point - *GPs need to learn more about the treatment options for strabismus.*

Dr Riva has shone a light on the psychological suffering attached to strabismus. No one can fail to empathise with the experiences described in our book, and touchingly portrayed in the photographs by Francesca and Remy. As I set out in No Joke, strabismus patients are often the butt of 'jokes' that are cruel and demeaning. This needs to stop and we believe that raising the profile of strabismus, ensuring that strabismus is taken more seriously, will help in this both directly and indirectly.

Action Point - *psychological support and measurement of their health associated with quality of life for strabismus patients should be combined with medical care.*

Through all of our discussions across the team, it has become clearer as to why strabismus is a neglected eye condition. We hope that this book has gone some way towards raising the profile of strabismus – but we want to achieve more than awareness, we hope this book can lead to positive change for strabismus sufferers everywhere.

And finally, if you are a strabismus sufferer yourself, we hope that this book has given you some comfort and support. Do not suffer in silence; there is help available, strabismus is not incurable.

Lucia and Francesca

MEET THE TEAM

LUCIA WILSON

Writer, co-creator and co-editor of Face to Face with Strabismus

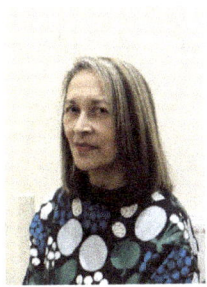

LUCIA WILSON is a British-born Anglo-Burmese writer of poetry, lyrics, and stories for all ages. She is a member of SACEM and PRS and lives in London. In 2019, The Adventures of Cedric the Bear was published (by Amsterdam Publishers), written by Lucia, illustrated by Anne Bowes, and co-created by Katie Eggington (the original designer of the physical bear). In this book, Lucia created a group of disabled characters (including the Pet Paralympians). As she discussed with Bridget Galton of the Ham & High newspaper, she is keen for children with disabilities to see themselves positively reflected in children's books.

Lucia's latest children's book is called Reggie Ruby, the Pirate of the Trees which features a boy with strabismus trying to protect the urban forest in London. Mr Saurabh Jain kindly advised her on the medical information related to strabismus.

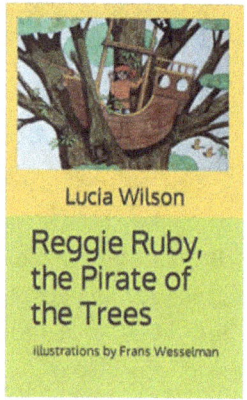

Other children's books by Lucia include

Costa the Cat in Corfu
Millie and the Pirate Moon

Lucia is also the author of The Karloff Tiara, a novella
www.luciawilson.co.uk

Francesca Cesari
Photographer, co-creator and co-editor of
Face to Face with Strabismus

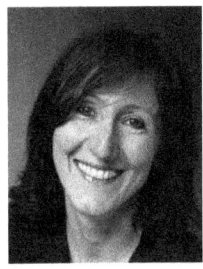

FRANCESCA CESARI
is an Italian photographer based in Bologna.
With an academic background in Art History, she started
as a self-taught photographer and perfected her skills
at the LCP in London.

Along with commercial assignments and teaching
photography she mainly works with long-term personal
projects, where her artistic research concentrates on
people, often portrayed in their environment with natural
light.
Her photography aims, above all, to observe human
relations and the fundamental passages of our existence;
in particular she has addressed the topics of family,
motherhood, adolescence, and human relationships, with
a focus on the feminine world.

A finalist for the Portraits-Hellerau Photography Award,
Photovisa, and Kuala Lumpur International Photoaward,
Francesca Cesari is the recipient of numerous

recognitions, including Honourable Mentions indifferent photography Awards (IPA, TIFA and JMCA). Her photographs have been featured in both personal and collective exhibitions, and her images are regularly published, both in Italy and abroad.

www.francescacesari.com

Mr Saurabh Jain

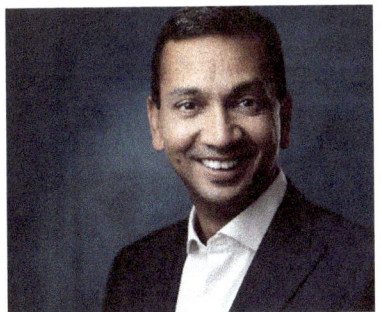

Saurabh Jain is a Consultant Ophthalmic Surgeon and the Clinical Director of Services at the Royal Free London NHS Trust in London and honorary consultant at UCLH, both large teaching hospitals in central London. He is an Honorary Associate Professor at UCL and the Senior personal Tutor for UCL medical school. He has special expertise in all aspects of Paediatric Ophthalmology, adult strabismus, toxin, and cataract surgery

He started his ophthalmology career at Kings College London. He was a specialist registrar at the Leicester royal Infirmary where he undertook further advanced training as a fellow in adult strabismus surgery. He also completed further specialist training in Paediatric Ophthalmology at the Manchester Royal Eye Hospital.

He is committed to teaching and training and has mentored several residents and fellows over the years. He has been awarded the Fellowship of the Higher Education Academy (FHEA) by University College London and the Fellowship of the European Board of Ophthalmology (FEBO). He runs two successful training courses annually: the London Eye Course and Binocular

He is a senior examiner for the Royal College of

Ophthalmologists, International Council of Ophthalmology, and the European Board of Ophthalmology.

He has a keen research interest in strabismus and ocular motility and has authored various research papers and textbook chapters. The findings from his research have been published in respected international ophthalmic journals, textbooks and presented at meetings worldwide. He has given several invited lectures worldwide. He is an active member of the Royal College of Ophthalmologists and the Education Officer for the British Isles Paediatric Ophthalmology and Strabismus Association. He has regularly refereed articles for the journals The British Journal of Ophthalmology, Strabismus, Eye and Ophthalmology.

He is involved in running a busy full-time clinical service at the Royal Free, Whittington and UCLH hospitals which includes clinical work, training junior surgeons and allied clinical professionals, research, and educational activities. His private practice is based at the Portland Hospital for Women and Children, London, and The London Clinic in Harley Street.

Dr Giovanni Battista Marcon

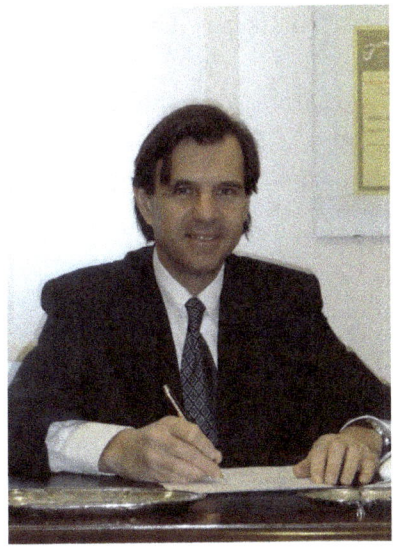

Dr Giovanni Battista Marcon was born in Aviano (PN) Italy in 1961. He graduated in Medicine at Padua University in 1985 and specialized in Ophthalmology (full marks and Laude) at the same University in 1989. He worked for about 10 years in the Ophthalmological Department of the Bassano del Grappa Public Hospital and then in 2000 became Head of the Ophthalmological department in the Public Hospital of Gorizia-Monfalcone (Italy).

In 2010 he left the Gorizia Hospital and founded the "Strabismus and Diplopia Centre" in Bassano del Grappa (Italy) of which he is the Director.

Dr Marcon is an Ophthalmic Surgeon. He has performed in his career more than 18,000 cataract surgeries, hundreds of glaucoma operations, retinal detachment surgeries and thousands of strabismus operations. Since

2010 he dedicated full time to the diagnosis and treatment of Child and Adult strabismus. He has been Secretary and President of the Italian Strabismological Association.

He serves as Secretary/Treasurer of the European Strabismological Association. (ESA) and of the International Pediatric Ophthalmology Strabismus Council (IPOSC).

Dr Marcon has participated as speaker in hundreds of National and International meetings. In many meetings, he has performed surgeries (live operations) mainly for cataract and strabismus surgeries.

From 1994 to 2010 he has been Head and Surgeon of the "Eye Rural Screening "at the North Kinangop Hospital in Naivasha (Kenya). For 15 years he went to Kenya twice a year for humanitarian purposes.

Dr Marcon is Author and Co-author of more than 100 scientific papers and co-author of 2 books in Italian. He has been a lecturer in many Strabismological Societies in Europe.

REMY HUNTER – Photographer

Remy Hunter is a professional headshot photographer of more than 20 years' experience based in London. He is a member of the Association of Professional Headshot Photographers and photographs actors, singers, dancers, writers, and anyone else needing headshots. His USP is working collaboratively with clients and directing from behind the camera in ways that feel comfortable for them.
You can see more of his work at www.remyhunterphotography.com

Remy provided excellent support to Francesca Cesari as our second photographer, producing the striking portraits of UK strabismus patient, Paul Boyce in a unique collaboration.

Dr. Silvia Riva

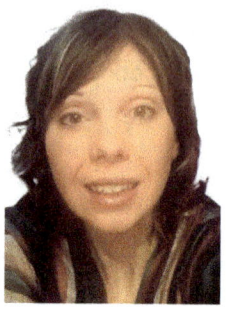

Silvia Riva is an Associate Professor of Psychology at St. Mary's University and a HCPC-registered clinical psychologist.

Silvia obtained a Bachelor degree in Psychology in 2003 and a Master Degree in Clinical Psychology in 2005 from the Catholic University of Sacred Heart in Milan (Italy). She obtained her PhD (Doctor Europaeus) from the Catholic University of Sacred Heart in Milan in 2012 investigating the use of heuristics and reasoning processes in medical choices.

Silvia's research interests concern decision processes under different conditions (stress, risk, uncertainty), as well as in several contexts (especially health care). In terms of theory, she is interested in how people make good decisions to improve their health-related quality of life and to cope with the challenges they face in their environment (e.g., diseases, stress, risks).

Furthermore, Silvia is a Registered Clinical Psychologist with the HCPC and a Certified Cognitive Behavioural

Therapist. Her approach is based on Acceptance and Commitment Therapy (ACT) as well as Rational Emotive Behaviour Therapy (REBT).

www.stmarys.ac.uk/staff-directory/silva-riva

www.dottorelondon.com/it/doctor/dott-ssa-silvia-riva/

Personal website: **www.silviariva.net/**